Book of Sayings

PETA ZAFIR

Book of Sayings

Book 3

©2021 Peta Zafir

All rights reserved.

No part of this book may be reproduced in any form or by any electronic or mechanical means, including information storage and retrieval systems, without written permission from the author, except in the case of a reviewer, who may quote brief passages embodied in critical articles or in a review.

Trademarked names appear throughout this book. Rather than use a trademark symbol with every occurrence of a trademarked name, names are used in an editorial fashion, with no intention of infringement of the respective owner's trademark.

The information in this book is distributed on an "as is" basis, without warranty. Although every precaution has been taken in the preparation of this work, neither the author nor the publisher shall have any liability to any person or entity with respect to any loss or damage caused or alleged to be caused directly or indirectly by the information contained in this book.

Peta Zafir Publishing
www.petazafir.com

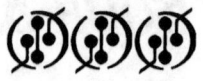

ISBN 978-0-6452140-5-5

Peta Zafir Publishing
www.petazafir.com
Peta Zafir You Tube Channel

BOOKS BY PETA ZAFIR
Health in Poetry Book 1
Health in Poetry Book 2
Book of Sayings Book 1
Book of Sayings Book 2
Book of Sayings Book 3
Book of Sayings Book 4
Scenar For Beginners

All books are available in print and eBook format from:
www.petazafir.com/books

Dedication

I dedicate this book to my second son, Anton who has taught me to be brave in my actions and to progress one step at a time. He illustrates this every day to me and others, through his compassion, training, sportsmanship, and his focus on excellence.

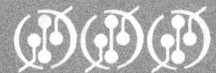

Book of Sayings   Book 3

Don't become tainted by others opinions
Don't conform to the pressure of society
Dance to your own tune

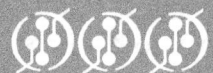

Book of Sayings   Book 3

The most valuable aspects in life

are given freely

Respect and cherish them

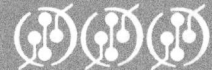

Book of Sayings   Book 3

Kindness done without expectation

brings its own reward

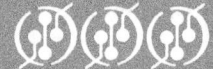

Book of Sayings   Book 3

Unlimited Possibilities

Your way

Your focus

Your understanding

No Limitations

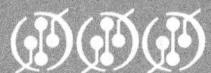

Book of Sayings   Book 3

You have the strength to Survive

Draw on it

You have the force to Fight

Develop it

You have the ability to Learn

Search for it

You have the right to Happiness

Never give up

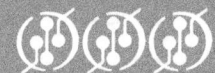

Book of Sayings   Book 3

Life happens
Work through the events of Past
Refine and Clear the Present and
Clarify the pathways of your Future

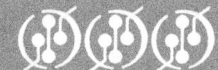

Book of Sayings   Book 3

Feel the pain

Work through it

Release it and

Step into a full happy healthy life

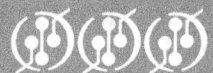

Book of Sayings   Book 3

Every decision

Opens up a new choice in life

Book of Sayings   Book 3

There is always a Path
Sometimes it needs to be illuminated

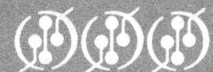

Book of Sayings   Book 3

Never lose focus
Some lessons are hard to bear
Yet important to learn

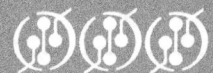

My strength embraces you
through your times of trouble and
My laughter shares with you
through your times of joy

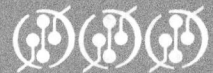

Book of Sayings   Book 3

My Past may explain
Why I act or
Have acted in a certain way
This is no longer an excuse
I use this as a point of growth
To change my present
And create my future

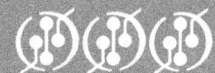

There comes a time in life when you
Accept your past
Assess the person you are
Make the changes you want
Evaluate daily your progress
Live fully in the present
Construct the foundations of your Future

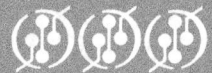

Book of Sayings   Book 3

You never realise the strength you have

until you need to draw on it

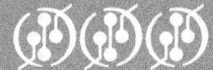

Book of Sayings   Book 3

Your body, mind and spirit will change
when your perception and beliefs change

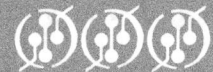

Book of Sayings   Book 3

Don't look back into a Past
that can't change
Don't look forward to a Future
that may change
Start in the Present
Where change can occur

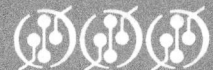

Book of Sayings   Book 3

Family is not only connection through Blood
Family are unconditionally loving and
A safe and peaceful Haven
Family is all encompassing

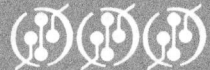

Book of Sayings   Book 3

May your choices be wise
Your friends be loyal
Your family be loving
Your work be rewarding
Your expenses be low
Your wages be high and
You find joy and happiness
Walking on the beach
Watching a sunset

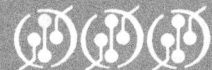

Book of Sayings   Book 3

Your Life Matters
Choose your friends wisely
Choose your food healthy
Choose your home safely
Choose your job happily
Choose your path adventurously

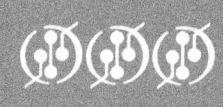

Life is too short to waste on people
who can't keep up with you
Don't be held back because
others don't travel your Path
Sometimes you need to walk alone

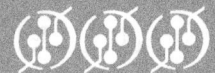

Book of Sayings   Book 3

Everything is possible

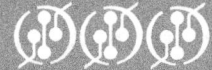

Book of Sayings   Book 3

Everyone has
A different way
A different focus and
A different understanding
Find your unique path

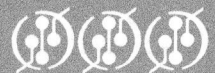

Book of Sayings Book 3

Don't limit yourself because of
Negative thoughts
Others comments
Environmental pressures and
Present situations
Chart your own course

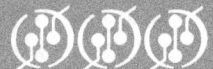

Book of Sayings   Book 3

Do the work
Clear the Baggage
Understand your gifts
And illuminate the person
you were born to be

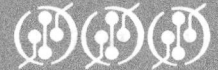

Book of Sayings   Book 3

We all have the strength to survive regardless of what we have experienced

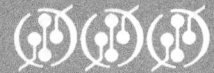

Follow your dreams
Do what is needed
Find the strength within
Trust in Yourself
And achieve your goals

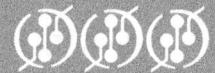

Book of Sayings   Book 3

People who say "It can't be done"
Speak from fear or jealousy
Believe in yourself, and step forward

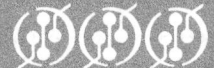

Book of Sayings   Book 3

Never let another person's comments define You

Their Perceptions may be defined by their own inadequacies

Based in fear, envy and jealousy

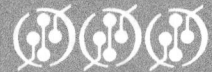

Life is an adventure
Live it
Feel it
Laugh in it
Cry through it
Experience it

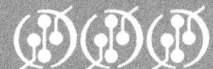

Book of Sayings   Book 3

Be Visible, Be Present

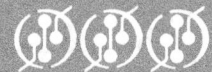

Book of Sayings   Book 3

When life becomes too complicated
Stand still and reflect
Consider your options then proceed
Simplicity is the way

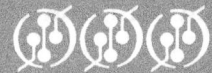

Book of Sayings   Book 3

Life is a Journey
Follow your intuition
Believe in your feelings
Find your focus
Direct yourself
Work with purpose and discipline
Live in integrity and
Trust in your life's destination

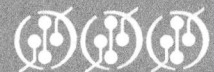

Book of Sayings   Book 3

Fear can overtake You
Fear can create health issues
Determine where it originates
Discover why it engulfs you
Develop awareness of its action
Harness your strength
Work through it, Then let it go and
Journey into Consciousness

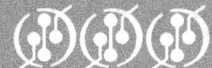

Book of Sayings   Book 3

In our society we value
Youth instead of Wisdom
Jeopardy instead of Intelligence
Money before Integrity
Sarcasm instead of Honesty
Criticism instead of Understanding
Hurt instead of Compassion
Isolation instead of Acceptance
Doubt instead of Trust
Pessimism instead of Optimism
Learn to Care

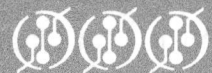

Book of Sayings　Book 3

Be brave enough to dream
Strong enough to act and
Creative enough to enjoy

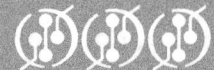

Parenthood

The most important role in life

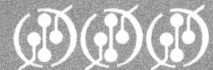

Family

are all living things that offer unconditional love

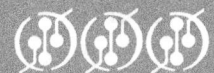

Life may place us on an unexpected path
of adversity, trials and tribulations
Draw on your strength to persevere
Become aware, clear the debris and rebuild,
This is what defines the person

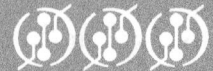

There are no spiritual limitations
Only those that you place on yourself
due to your beliefs
and internal messages

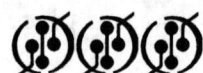

Peta Zafir Publishing
www.petazafir.com
Peta Zafir You Tube Channel

BOOKS BY PETA ZAFIR

Health in Poetry Book 1
Health in Poetry Book 2
Book of Sayings Book 1
Book of Sayings Book 2
Book of Sayings Book 3
Book of Sayings Book 4
Scenar For Beginners

All books are available in print and eBook format from:
www.petazafir.com/books

Notes

NOTES

Notes

www.ingramcontent.com/pod-product-compliance
Lightning Source LLC
Chambersburg PA
CBHW071835290426
44109CB00017B/1829